Pescatarian Recipe Book

A Complete set of Seafood and Green Recipes for a Healthy Life!

Lara Dillard

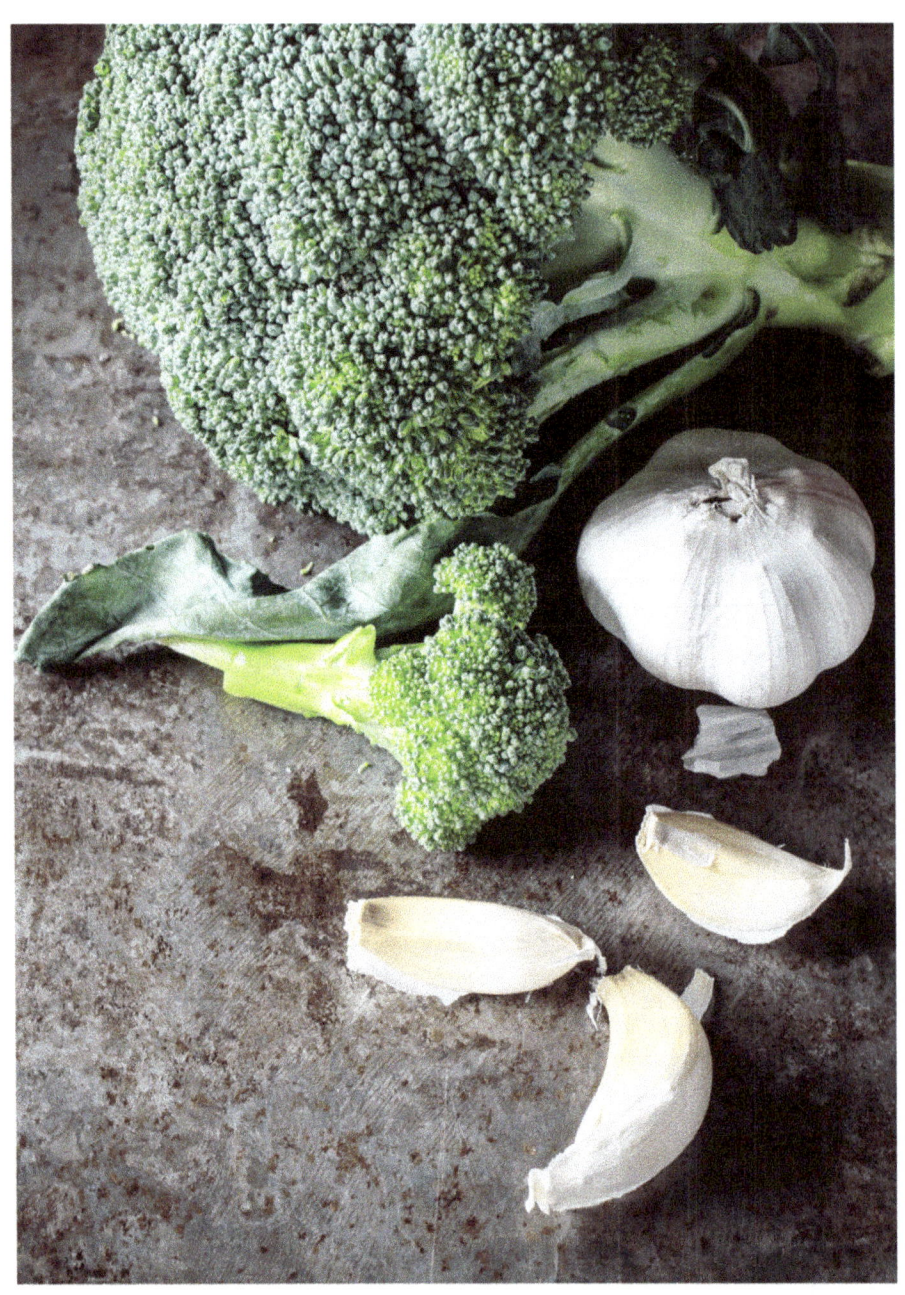

© copyright 2021 – all rights reserved.

the content contained within this book may not be reproduced, duplicated or transmitted without direct written permission from the author or the publisher.

under no circumstances will any blame or legal responsibility be held against the publisher, or author, for any damages, reparation, or monetary loss due to the information contained within this book. either directly or indirectly.

legal notice:

this book is copyright protected. this book is only for personal use. you cannot amend, distribute, sell, use, quote or paraphrase any part, or the content within this book, without the consent of the author or publisher.

disclaimer notice:

please note the information contained within this document is for educational and entertainment purposes only. all effort has been executed to present accurate, up to date, and reliable, complete information. no warranties of any kind are declared or implied. readers acknowledge that the author is not engaging in the rendering of legal, financial, medical or professional advice. the content within this book has been derived from various sources. please consult a licensed professional before attempting any techniques outlined in this book.

by reading this document, the reader agrees that under no circumstances is the author responsible for any losses, direct or indirect, which are incurred as a result of the use of information contained within this document, including, but not limited to, — errors, omissions, or inaccuracies.

Table of Contents

Broccoli and Garlic 6
Mustard Glazed Carrots 8
Garlic Artichokes 10
Farro Side Dish 12
Flavored Polenta 14
Pressure Pot Peanuts 17
Stuffed Mushrooms 20
Mashed Ruby Yams 22
Saucy Sweet Potatoes with Zucchini and Peppers 24
Herbed Potatoes with Mediterranean Dipping Sauce 27
Roma Tomato Bites with Halloumi Cheese 30
Spicy Winter Squash Bites 33
Butter Squash Fritters 36
Herbed Roasted Potatoes 38
Indian-Style Garnet Sweet Potatoes 40
Easy Frizzled Leeks 42
Easy Sautéed Green Beans 44
Colby Potato Patties 47
Smoked Veggie Omelet 49
Sweet Potato and Carrot Croquettes 51
Manchego and Potato Patties 53
Mint-Butter Stuffed Mushrooms 55
Basic Pepper French Fries 57
Pantano Romanesco with Vegan Cheese Appetizer 59
Winter Sausage with Root Vegetables 61
Fried Catfish 63
Lemony Vegan Salmon 66

SALMON OMELET	68
GOLDEN COD FISH NUGGETS	70
FULL BAKED TROUT EN PAPILLOTE WITH HERBS	72
BREADED SCALLOPS	74
HOT SALMON AND BROCCOLI	77
SOY SAUCE GLAZED COD	79
COUNTY BAKED CRAB CAKES	81
AIR FRIED SALMON	83
AIR FRIED DRAGON SHRIMP	85
CHEESY HADDOCK	87
FOIL BAKED SALMON	89
PASTA WITH CAPERS AND TUNA	92
TUNA BOWLS	95
RANCH FISH FILLET	97
PAPRIKA SALMON	99
FISH STICKS	101
FISH FILLET WITH PESTO SAUCE	103
HOT CRISPY PRAWNS	105

Broccoli and Garlic

Servings: 4

Total Time: 22 Minutes

Calories: 182

Fat: 4 g

Protein: 6 g

Carbs: 6 g

Fiber: 2 g

Ingredients and Quantity

- 1/2 cup water
- 1 tbsp. olive oil
- 6 garlic cloves, minced
- 1 broccoli head, florets separated
- 1 tbsp. rice wine
- A pinch salt and black pepper

Direction

1. Put the water in your Pressure pot. Add steamer basket and then put the broccoli inside.
2. Cover and cook on High for 10 minutes.
3. Transfer broccoli to a bowl filled with cold water.
4. Leave aside for a few minutes. Then drain and put in another bowl.
5. Clean your Pressure pot and set the pot on Sauté mode.
6. Add oil and heat it up. Add garlic, stir and cook for 1 minute.
7. Add broccoli, salt, pepper and rice wine.
8. Stir, cover pot, cook on High for 1 minute more.
9. Divide amongst plates and serve. Enjoy!

Mustard Glazed Carrots

Servings: 4

Total Time: 30 Minutes

Calories: 200

Fat: 4 g

Protein: 6 g

Carbs: 9 g

Fiber: 7 g

Ingredients and Quantity

- 1/4 tsp. baking soda
- 1 tsp. thyme, dried
- 1 tbsp. mustard
- 1 tbsp. olive oil
- 3 pounds carrots, cut into medium strips
- 1 tbsp. maple syrup

- 2 tbsp. veggie stock

Direction

1. Set your Pressure pot on Sauté mode. Add oil and heat up.
2. Add maple syrup, mustard, baking soda and veggie stock.
3. Stir and cook for 1 minute.
4. Add carrots and thyme. Stir a bit.
5. Cover and cook on High for 4 minutes.
6. Divide amongst plates. Serve and enjoy!

Garlic Artichokes

Servings: 2

Total Time: 17 Minutes

Calories: 173

Fat: 6 g

Protein: 9 g

Carbs: 6 g

Fiber: 2 g

Ingredients and Quantity

- 4 artichokes, trimmed and stems removed
- 4 tsp. olive oil
- 1/2 cup veggie stock
- 2 tsp. garlic, minced
- A pinch salt

Direction

1. Put the artichokes in your Pressure pot. Add garlic, a pinch of salt and oil. Toss them a bit.
2. Add the stock, cover the pot and cook on High for 7 minutes.
3. Divide amongst plates. Serve and enjoy!

Farro Side Dish

Servings: 4

Total Time: 50 Minutes

Calories: 152

Fat: 3 g

Protein: 5 g

Carbs: 7 g

Fiber: 4 g

Ingredients and Quantity

- 1 tsp. lemon juice
- A pinch salt and black pepper
- 1 cup cherries, pitted
- 10 mint leaves, chopped
- 1 tbsp. balsamic vinegar
- 1 cup faro

- 3 cups water
- 1 tbsp. olive oil
- 1/4 cup chives, chopped

Direction

1. Put farro and water in your Pressure pot. Cover and cook on High for 40 minutes.
2. Drain the farro and transfer to a bowl.
3. Add vinegar, oil, lemon juice, salt, pepper, cherries, mint and chives.
4. Toss well and divide amongst plates. Serve and enjoy!

Flavored Polenta

Servings: 6

Total Time: 17 Minutes

Calories: 100

Fat: 1 g

Protein: 2 g

Carbs: 10 g

Fiber: 2 g

Ingredients and Quantity

- 1/3 cup sun-dried tomatoes, chopped
- 2 tbsp. olive oil
- 1/2 cup onion, chopped
- 2 tsp. oregano, chopped
- 1 tsp. rosemary, chopped
- 1 cup polenta

- 1 bay leaf
- A pinch salt
- 4 cups veggie stock
- 2 tsp. garlic, minced
- 2 tbsp. parsley, chopped
- 3 tbsp. basil, chopped

Direction

1. Set your Pressure pot on sauté mode. Add oil and heat it up.
2. Add onion, stir and cook for 1 minute.
3. Add garlic, stir and cook for 1 minute more.
4. Add sun-dried tomatoes, stock, salt, bay leaf, rosemary, oregano, half of the parsley, half of the basil and the polenta.
5. Stir, cover and cook on High for 5 minutes.
6. Discard bay leaf, stir polenta, add the rest of the basil and parsley.
7. Leave everything aside for a few minutes more.

8. Divide amongst plates and serve. Enjoy!

Pressure Pot Peanuts

Servings: 4

Total Time: 1 Hour 20 Minutes

Calories: 120

Fat: 5 g

Protein: 6 g

Carbs: 10 g

Fiber: 3 g

Ingredients and Quantity

- 3 garlic cloves
- 1 tbsp. palm sugar
- 1 pound raw peanuts, rinsed well
- 3 cinnamon sticks
- 3 tbsp. salt
- star anise

- 4 red hot chili peppers

Direction

1. Put peanuts in your Pressure pot. Add water to cover, cinnamon stick, salt, anise, sugar and chili pepper.
2. Stir, cover and cook on High for 1 hour and 20 minutes.
3. Release pressure naturally. Leave aside for 20 minutes.
4. Transfer the peanuts to a serving bowl. Serve and enjoy!

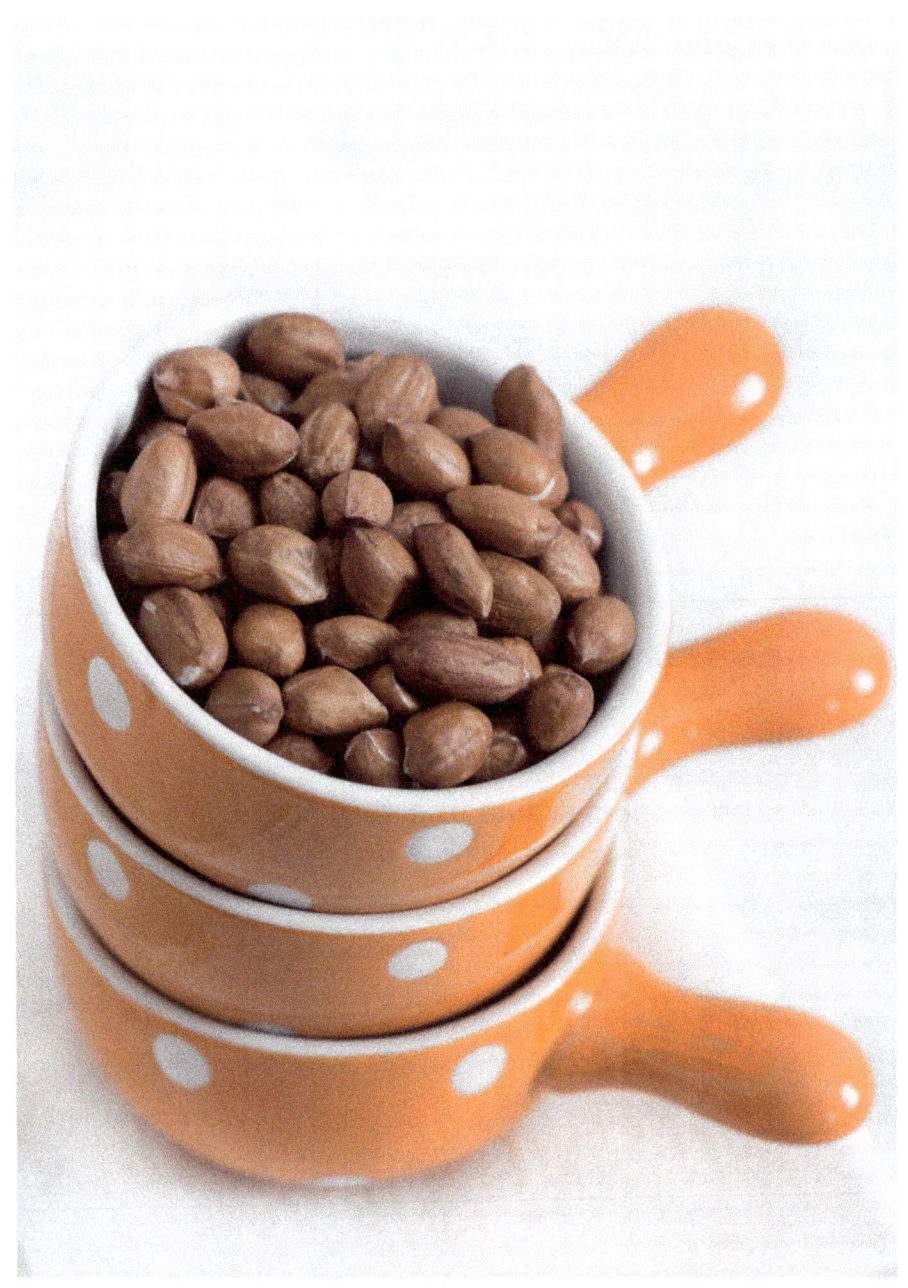

Stuffed Mushrooms

Servings: 2

Total Time: 16 Minutes

Calories: 176

Fat: 14.7 g

Protein: 6 g

Carbs: 10.5 g

Fiber: 4 g

Ingredients and Quantity

- 2 tsp. cumin powder
- 4 garlic cloves, peeled and minced
- 1 small onion, peeled and chopped
- 2 tbsp. bran cereal, crushed
- 18 medium-sized white mushrooms

- Fine sea salt and freshly ground black pepper, to your taste
- A pinch ground allspice
- 2 tbsp. olive oil

Direction

1. First, clean the mushrooms; remove the middle stalks from the mushrooms to prepare the "shells".
2. Grab a mixing dish and thoroughly combine the remaining items.
3. Fill the mushrooms with the prepared mixture.
4. Cook the mushrooms at 345 degrees F heat for 12 minutes. Enjoy!

Mashed Ruby Yams

Servings: 4

Total Time: 20 Minutes

Calories: 223

Fat: 14.7 g

Protein: 4.8 g

Carbs: 18.6 g

Fiber: 5 g

Ingredients and Quantity

- 1/3 cup maple syrup
- 2 eggs, beaten
- 1/2 tsp. ground black pepper
- 1 tsp. cayenne pepper
- 1/3 cup extra virgin olive oil
- 1 1/2 tsp. pink Himalayan salt flakes

- 5 ruby yams, peeled
- 1 1/2 tbsp. coconut cream

Direction

1. Boil ruby yams until they're fork tender.
2. Then, combine all the remaining ingredients using an electric mixer or a wire whisk.
3. Scrape the mixture into a baking dish.
4. Transfer the baking dish to the air fryer and bake for 20 minutes at 305 degrees F. Serve and enjoy!

Saucy Sweet Potatoes with Zucchini and Peppers

Servings: 4

Total Time: 20 Minutes **Calories:** 225

Fat: 12.9 g

Protein: 2.8 g

Carbs: 27.3 g

Fiber: 4 g

Ingredients and Quantity

- 1/4 cup olive oil
- 1 Serrano pepper, deveined and thinly sliced
- 1 bell pepper, deveined and thinly sliced
- 2 large-sized sweet potatoes, peeled and quartered
- 1 to 2 carrots, cut into matchsticks

- 1 1/2 tbsp. maple syrup
- 1/2 tsp. porcini powder
- 1/4 tsp. mustard powder
- 1/2 tsp. fennel seeds
- 1 medium-sized zucchini, sliced
- 1 tbsp. garlic powder
- 1/4 tsp. ground black pepper
- 1/2 tsp. fine sea salt
- Tomato ketchup, for serving

Direction

1. Place the sweet potatoes, zucchini, peppers and the carrot into the air fryer cooking basket.
2. Drizzle with olive oil and toss to coat; cook in the preheated machine at 355 degrees F for 14 minutes.
3. While the vegetables are cooking, prepare the sauce by thoroughly whisking the other ingredients, without the tomato ketchup.

4. Lightly grease a baking dish that fits into your machine.

5. Transfer cooked vegetables to the prepared baking dish; add the sauce and toss to coat well.

6. Turn the machine to 395 degrees F and cook the vegetables for 4 more minutes.

7. Serve warm with tomato ketchup on the side. Enjoy!

Herbed Potatoes with Mediterranean Dipping Sauce

Servings: 4

Total Time: 20 Minutes

Calories: 303

Fat: 12.2 g

Protein: 8.5 g

Carbs: 37.3 g

Fiber: 3.1 g

Ingredients and Quantity

- 2 pounds Russet potatoes, peeled and cubed
- 1 1/2 tbsp. melted almond butter
- 1 tsp. sea salt flakes
- 1 sprig rosemary, leaves only, crushed

- 2 sprigs thyme, leaves only, crushed
- 1/2 tsp. freshly cracked black peppercorns

For the Mediterranean Dipping Sauce:

- 1/2 cup vegan cheese
- 1/3 cup yogurt
- 1 tbsp. freshly dill, chopped
- 1 tbsp. olive oil

Direction

1. Firstly, set your Air Fryer to cook at 360 degrees F.
2. Now, add the potato cubes to the bowl with cold water and soak them approximately for 33 minutes.
3. After that, dry the potato cubes using a paper towel.

4. In a mixing dish, thoroughly whisk the melted butter with sea salt flakes, rosemary, thyme, and freshly cracked peppercorns.

5. Rub the potato cubes with this butter/spice mix.

6. Air-fry the potato cubes in the cooking basket for 17 to 20 minutes or until cooked through; make sure to shake the potatoes to cook them evenly.

7. Meanwhile, make the Mediterranean dipping sauce by mixing the remaining ingredients.

8. Serve warm potatoes with Mediterranean sauce for dipping. Enjoy!

Roma Tomato Bites with Halloumi Cheese

Servings: 4

Total Time: 20 Minutes

Calories: 428

Fat: 38.4 g

Protein: 18.8 g

Carbs: 4.5 g

Fiber: 2.2 g

Ingredients and Quantity

For the Sauce:

- 1/3 cup extra-virgin olive oil
- 1/2 cup vegan cheese, grated
- 1 tsp. garlic puree

- 1/2 tsp. fine sea salt
- 4 tbsp. pecans, chopped

For the Tomato Bites:

- 2 large sized Roma tomatoes, cut into thin slices and pat them dry
- 8 oz. vegan cheese, cut into thin slices
- 1 tsp. dried basil
- 1/4 tsp. red pepper flakes, crushed
- 1/8 tsp. sea salt
- 1/3 cup onions, sliced
- 1 tsp. dried basil

Direction

1. Start by preheating your air fryer to 380 F.
2. Make the sauce by mixing all ingredients, except the extra-virgin olive oil, in your food processor.

3. While the machine is running, slowly and gradually pour in the olive oil; puree until everything is well - blended.
4. Now, spread 1 teaspoon of the sauce over the top of each tomato slice.
5. Place a slice of vegan cheese on each tomato slice.
6. Top with onion slices. Sprinkle with basil, red pepper, and sea salt.
7. Transfer the bites to the Air Fryer basket.
8. Drizzle with olive oil and cook for approximately 14 minutes.
9. Arrange these bites on a nice serving platter, garnish with the remaining sauce and serve at room temperature. Enjoy!

Spicy Winter Squash Bites

Servings: 8

Total Time: 23 Minutes

Calories: 113

Fat: 3 g

Protein: 1.6 g

Carbs: 22.6 g

Fiber: 2 g

Ingredients and Quantity

- 2 tsp. fresh mint leaves, chopped
- 1/3 cup brown sugar
- 1 1/2 tsp. red pepper chili flakes
- 2 tbsp. melted almond butter
- 3 pounds winter squash, peeled, seeded and cubed

Direction

1. Toss all of the above ingredients in a large-sized mixing dish.

2. Roast the squash bites for 30 minutes at 325 degrees F in your Air Fryer, turning once or twice.

3. Serve with a homemade dipping sauce. Enjoy!

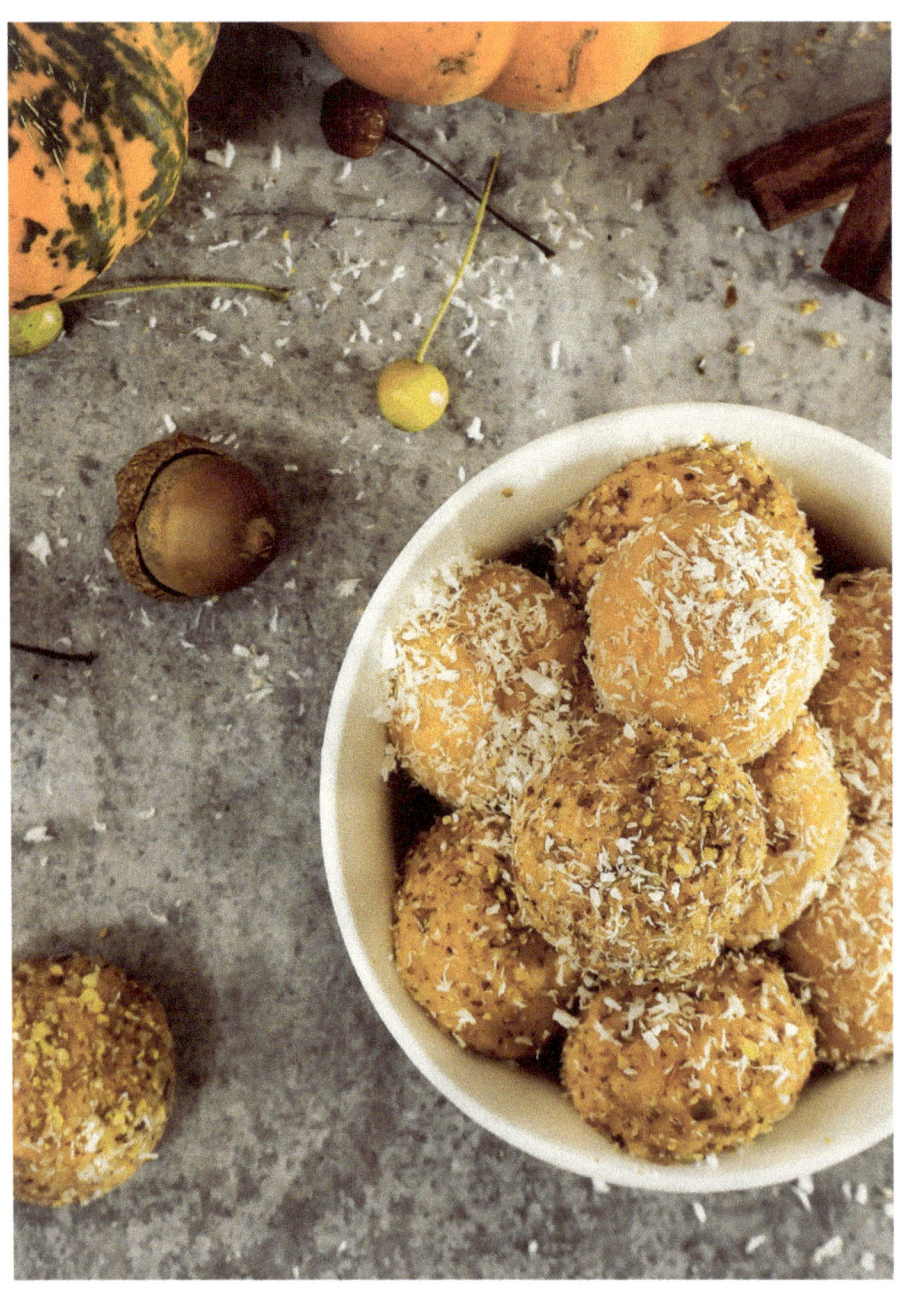

Butter Squash Fritters

Servings: 4

Total Time: 22 Minutes

Calories: 152

Fat: 10 g

Protein: 5.8 g

Carbs: 9.4 g

Fiber: 1.3 g

Ingredients and Quantity

- 1/3 cup all-purpose flour
- 1/3 tsp. freshly ground black pepper, or more, to taste 1/3 tsp. dried sage
- 4 garlic cloves, minced
- 1 1/2 tbsp. olive oil
- 1/3 butternut squash, peeled and grated 2 eggs,

well whisked 1 tsp. fine sea salt
- A pinch ground allspice

Direction

1. Thoroughly combine all ingredients in a mixing bowl.
2. Preheat your air fryer to 345 degrees and set the timer for 17 minutes; cook until your fritters are browned.
3. Serve right away. Enjoy!

Herbed Roasted Potatoes

Servings: 4

Total Time: 24 Minutes

Calories: 208

Fat: 7.1 g

Protein: 3.6 g

Carbs: 33.8 g

Fiber: 3 g

Ingredients and Quantity

- 1 tsp. crushed, dried thyme
- 1 tsp. ground black pepper
- 2 tbsp. olive oil
- 1/2 tbsp. crushed, dried rosemary
- 3 potatoes, peeled, washed and cut into wedges
- 1/2 tsp. seasoned salt

Direction

1. Lay the potatoes in the air fryer cooking basket, drizzle olive oil over your potatoes.
2. Then, cook for 17 minutes at 353 degrees F.
3. Toss with the seasonings and serve warm with your favorite salad on the side. Enjoy!

Indian-Style Garnet Sweet Potatoes

Servings: 4

Total Time: 24 Minutes

Calories: 103

Fat: 9.1 g

Protein: 1.9 g

Carbs: 4.9 g

Fiber: 1.2 g

Ingredients and Quantity

- 1/3 tsp. white pepper
- 1 tbsp. almond butter, melted
- 1/2 tsp. turmeric powder
- 5 garnet sweet potatoes, peeled and diced

- 11/2 tbsp. maple syrup
- 2 tsp. tamarind paste
- 1 1/2 tbsp. fresh lime juice
- 1 1/2 tsp. ground allspice

Direction

1. In a mixing bowl, toss all ingredients until sweet potatoes are well coated.
2. Air-fry them at 335 degrees F for 12 minutes.
3. Pause the air fryer and toss again.
4. Increase the temperature to 390 degrees F and cook for an additional 10 minutes.
5. Eat warm. Enjoy!

Easy Frizzled Leeks

Servings: 6

Total Time: 52 Minutes

Calories: 291

Fat: 6 g

Protein: 5.7 g

Carbs: 53.3 g

Fiber: 4.3 g

Ingredients and Quantity

- 1/2 tsp. porcini powder
- 1 1/2 cup rice flour
- 1 tbsp. vegetable oil
- 3 medium-sized leeks, sliced into julienne strips
- 2 large-sized dishes with ice water
- 2 tsp. onion powder

- Fine sea salt and cayenne pepper, to taste

Direction

1. Allow the leeks to soak in ice water for about 25 minutes; drain well.
2. Place the rice flour, salt, cayenne pepper, onions powder, and porcini powder into a resealable bag.
3. Add the celery and shake to coat well.
4. Drizzle vegetable oil over the seasoned leeks.
5. Air fry at 390 degrees F for about 18 minutes; turn them halfway through the cooking time.
6. Serve with homemade mayonnaise or any other sauce for dipping. Enjoy!

Easy Sautéed Green Beans

Servings: 4

Total Time: 12 Minutes

Calories: 53

Fat: 3 g

Protein: 1.6 g

Carbs: 6.1 g

Fiber: 1.2 g

Ingredients and Quantity

- 3/4 pound green beans, cleaned
- 1 tbsp. balsamic vinegar
- 1/4 tsp. kosher salt
- 1/2 tsp. mixed peppercorns, freshly cracked
- 1 tbsp. almond butter
- Sesame seeds, to serve

Direction

1. Set your air fryer to cook at 390 F.
2. Mix the green beans with all of the above ingredients, apart from the sesame seeds.
3. Set the timer for 10 minutes.
4. Meanwhile, toast the sesame seeds in a small-sized nonstick skillet; make sure to stir continuously.
5. Serve sautéed green beans on a nice serving platter sprinkled with toasted sesame seeds. Enjoy!

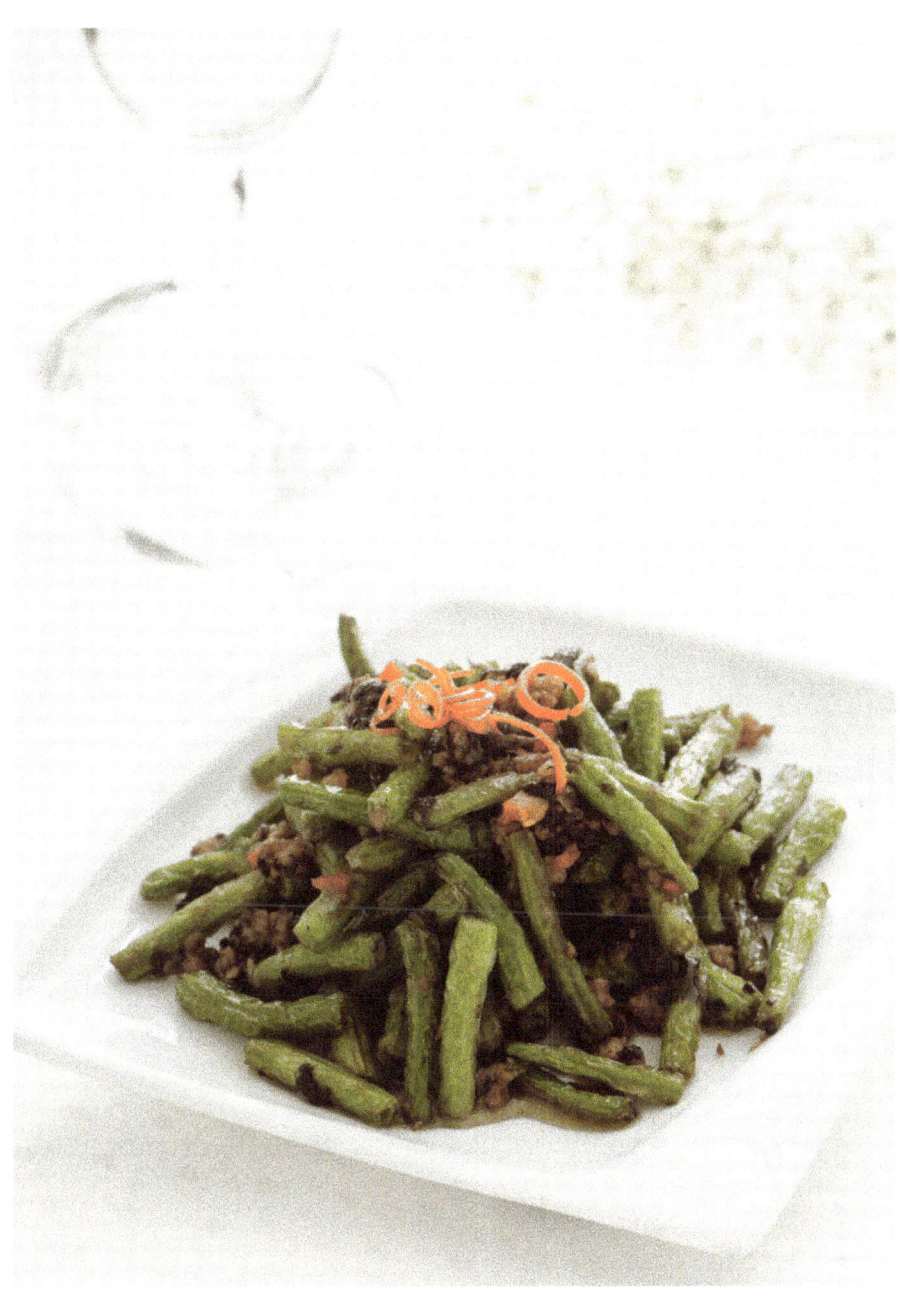

Colby Potato Patties

Servings: 8

Total Time: 15 Minutes

Calories: 291

Fat: 18 g

Protein: 9.3 g

Carbs: 23.7 g

Fiber: 1.7 g

Ingredients and Quantity

- 2 pounds white potatoes, peeled and grated 1/2 cup scallions, finely chopped
- 1/2 tsp. freshly ground black pepper, or more, to taste
- 1 tbsp. fine sea salt
- 1/2 tsp. hot paprika

- 2 cups vegan cheese, shredded
- 1/4 cup canola oil
- 1 cup crushed crackers

Direction

1. Firstly, boil the potatoes until fork tender.
2. Drain, peel and mash your potatoes.
3. Thoroughly mix the mashed potatoes with scallions, pepper, salt, paprika, and cheese.
4. Then, shape the balls using your hands.
5. Now, flatten the balls to make the patties.
6. In a shallow bowl, mix canola oil with crushed crackers.
7. Roll the patties over the crumb mixture.
8. Next, cook your patties at 360 degrees F approximately 10 minutes, working in batches.
9. Serve with tabasco mayo if desired. Enjoy!

Smoked Veggie Omelet

Servings: 2

Total Time: 14 Minutes

Calories: 226

Fat: 11.5 g

Protein: 16.3 g

Carbs: 14.2 g

Fiber: 5 g

Ingredients and Quantity

- 1/3 cup cherry tomatoes, chopped
- 1 bell pepper, seeded and chopped
- 1/3 tsp. freshly ground black pepper
- 1/2 purple onion, peeled and sliced
- 1 tsp. smoked cayenne pepper
- 15 tbsp. apple sauce

- 1/3 cup smoked tofu, crumbled
- 1 tsp. seasoned salt
- 1 1/2 tbsp. fresh chives, chopped

Direction

1. Brush a baking dish with a spray coating.
2. Throw all ingredients, minus fresh chives, into the baking dish; give it a good stir.
3. Cook about 15 minutes at 325 degrees F.
4. Garnish with fresh chopped chives. Serve and enjoy!

Sweet Potato and Carrot Croquettes

Servings: 4

Total Time: 22 Minutes

Calories: 206

Fat: 5 g

Protein: 8.3 g

Carbs: 32 g

Fiber: 2.1 g

Ingredients and Quantity

- 1/3 cup Swiss cheese, grated
- 1/3 tsp. fine sea salt
- 1/3 tsp. baking powder
- 1/3 cup scallions, finely chopped

- 3 carrots, trimmed and grated
- 1/2 tsp. freshly cracked black pepper
- 3 sweet potatoes, grated
- 1/3 cup all-purpose flour
- 6 tbsp. apple sauce

Direction

1. Place grated sweet potatoes and carrots on a paper towel and pat them dry.
2. Combine the potatoes and carrots with the other ingredients in the order listed above.
3. Then, create the balls using 1½ tablespoons of the vegetable mixture.
4. Then, gently flatten each ball.
5. Spritz the croquettes with a nonstick cooking oil.
6. Bake your croquettes for 13 minutes at 305 degrees F; work with batches.
7. Serve warm with tomato ketchup and mayonnaise. Enjoy!

Manchego and Potato Patties

Servings: 8

Total Time: 15 Minutes

Calories: 191

Fat: 8.7 g

Protein: 7 g

Carbs: 22 g

Fiber: 1.4 g

Ingredients and Quantity

- 1 cup vegan cheese, shredded
- 1 tsp. paprika
- 1 tsp. freshly ground black pepper
- 1/2 tbsp. fine sea salt

- 2 cups scallions, finely chopped
- 2 pounds Russet potatoes, peeled and grated
- 2 tbsp. canola oil
- 2 tsp. dried basil

Direction

1. Thoroughly combine all of the above ingredients.
2. Then, shape the balls using your hands.
3. Now, flatten the balls to make the patties.
4. Next, cook your patties at 360 degrees F approximately 10 minutes. Serve and enjoy!

Mint-Butter Stuffed Mushrooms

Servings: 3

Total Time: 20 Minutes

Calories: 290

Fat: 14.7 g

Protein: 28 g

Carbs: 13.4 g

Fiber: 3.3 g

Ingredients and Quantity

- 3 garlic cloves, minced
- 1 tsp. ground black pepper, or more, to taste 1/3 cup seasoned breadcrumbs
- 1 1/2 tbsp. fresh mint, chopped

- 1 tsp. salt, or more, to taste
- 1 1/2 tbsp. melted almond butter
- 14 medium-sized mushrooms, cleaned, stalks removed

Direction

1. Mix all of the above ingredients, minus the mushrooms, in a mixing bowl to prepare the filling.
2. Then, stuff the mushrooms with the prepared filling.
3. Air-fry stuffed mushrooms at 375 degrees F for about 12 minutes.
4. Taste for doneness and serve at room temperature as a vegetarian appetizer. Enjoy!

Basic Pepper French Fries

Servings: 4

Total Time: 33 Minutes

Calories: 263

Fat: 9.1 g

Protein: 4.5 g

Carbs: 42 g

Fiber: 3 g

Ingredients and Quantity

- 1/2 tsp. freshly ground black pepper
- 2 1/2 tbsp. canola oil
- 6 Russet potatoes, cut them into fries
- 1/2 tsp. crushed red pepper flakes

Direction

1. Start by preheating your air fryer to 340 degrees F.
2. Place the fries in your air fryer and toss them with the oil.
3. Add the seasonings and toss again.
4. Cook for 30 minutes, shaking your fries several times.
5. Taste for doneness and eat warm. Enjoy!

Pantano Romanesco with Vegan Cheese Appetizer

Servings: 4

Total Time: 20 Minutes

Calories: 237

Fat: 20.4 g

Protein: 13 g

Carbs: 0.9 g

Fiber: 0.9 g

Ingredients and Quantity

- 6 oz. vegan cheese, sliced
- 2 shallots, thinly sliced
- 2 Pantano Romanesco tomatoes, cut into 1/2 inch slices

- 1 1/2 tbsp. extra virgin olive oil
- 3/4 tsp. sea salt
- Fresh parsley, for garnish
- Fresh basil, chopped

Direction

1. Preheat your air fryer to 380 degrees F.
2. Now, pat each tomato slice dry using a paper towel.
3. Sprinkle each slice with salt and chopped basil.
4. Top with a slice of vegan cheese.
5. Top with the shallot slices; drizzle with olive oil.
6. Add the prepared tomato and feta "bites" to the air fryer food basket.
7. Cook in the air fryer for about 14 minutes.
8. Lastly, adjust seasonings to taste and serve garnished with fresh parsley leaves. Enjoy!

Winter Sausage with Root Vegetables

Servings: 4

Total Time: 30 Minutes

Calories: 289

Fat: 13.6 g

Protein: 13.3 g

Carbs: 32.5 g

Fiber: 6.7 g

Ingredients and Quantity

- 1/2 pound Italian sausage
- 3 sprigs rosemary
- medium-sized parsnip, sliced
- 1/3 pound fingerling potatoes

- 3 sprigs thyme
- 1/3 pounds carrots, trimmed and cut into matchsticks
- 1/2 celery stalk, sliced
- 2 garlic cloves, smashed
- 2 tbsp. extra-virgin olive oil
- 3 small-sized leeks, cut into halves lengthwise A pinch grated nutmeg
- Salt and black pepper, to taste

Direction

1. Arrange fingerling potatoes, carrots, celery, parsnip, and leeks on the bottom of the air fryer baking dish.
2. Tuck the garlic cloves around the vegetables.
3. Sprinkle with the seasonings and top with the sausage.
4. Roast approximately 33 minutes at 375 degrees F, stirring occasionally. Serve and enjoy!

Fried Catfish

Servings: 4

Total Time: 60 Minutes

Calories: 208

Fat: 9 g

Protein: 17 g

Carbs: 8 g

Fiber: 0.6 g

Ingredients and Quantity

- 4 catfish fillets
- 1/4 cup seasoned fish fry (I used Louisiana)
- 1 tbsp. olive oil
- 1 tbsp. parsley, chopped, optional

Direction

1. Preheat air fryer to 400F.
2. Rinse the catfish and pat dry.
3. Pour the fish fry seasoning in a large Ziploc bag.
4. Add the catfish to the bag, one at a time. Seal the bag and shake. Ensure the entire filet is coated with seasoning.
5. Spray olive oil on the top of each filet.
6. Place the filet in the air fryer basket (due to the size of my fillets, I cooked each one at a time). Close and cook for 10 minutes.
7. Flip the fish. Cook for an additional 10 minutes.
8. Flip the fish. Cook for an additional 2-3 minutes or until desired crispness.
9. 10.Top with parsley. Serve and enjoy!

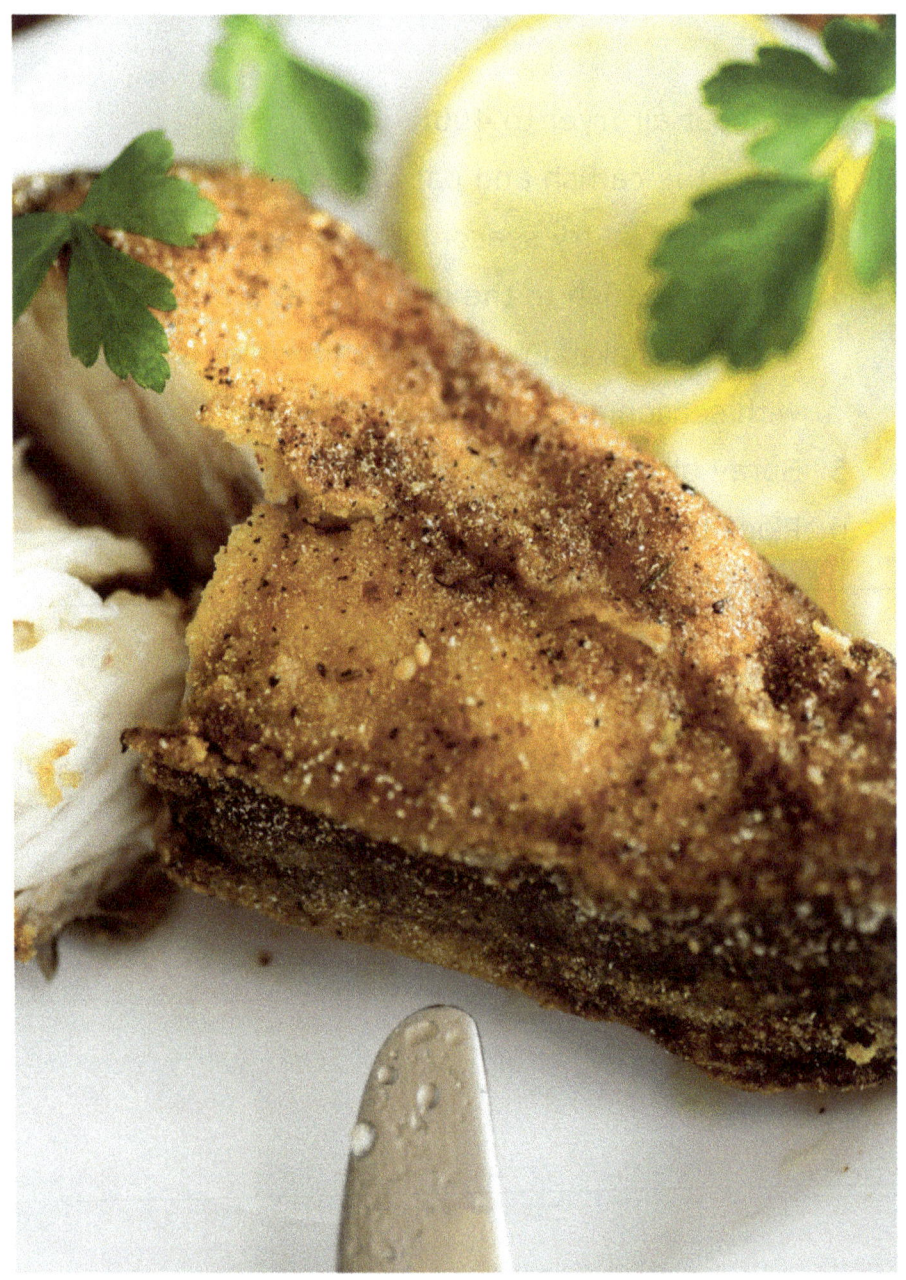

Lemony Vegan Salmon

Servings: 4

Total Time: 35 Minutes

Calories: 290

Fat: 16 g

Protein: 33 g

Carbs: 4 g

Fiber: 1 g

Ingredients and Quantity

- 2 tbsp. butter, melted
- 2 tbsp. green onions, sliced thinly
- 3/4 cup breadcrumbs, white, fresh
- 1/4 tsp. thyme leaves, dried
- 1 1/4 pounds salmon fillet, 1 piece
- 1/4 tsp. salt

- 1/4 cup vegan cheese, grated
- 2 tsp. lemon peel, grated

Direction

1. Preheat the air fryer at 350 degrees Fahrenheit.
2. Mist cooking spray onto a baking pan (shallow). Fill with pat-dried salmon.
3. Brush salmon with butter (1 tablespoon) before sprinkling with salt.
4. Combine the breadcrumbs with onions, thyme, lemon peel, cheese, and remaining butter (1 tablespoon).
5. Cover salmon with the breadcrumb mixture. Air-fry for fifteen totwenty-five minutes. Serve and enjoy!

Salmon Omelet

Servings: 2

Total Time: 18 Minutes

Calories: 193

Fat: 12.2 g

Protein: 19 g

Carbs: 1.3 g

Fiber: 0.1 g

Ingredients and Quantity

- 3 oz. smoked salmon, chopped
- 12 tbsp. apple sauce
- 1 tsp. scallions
- 1 pinch salt
- 1/4 tsp. ground black pepper
- 1/4 tsp. chili flakes
- 1/2 tsp. almond butter

- 2 tbsp. cream

Direction

1. Pour the apple sauce in a bowl.
2. Add the scallions and salt.
3. After this, sprinkle the apple sauce with the ground black pepper, chili flakes and cream.
4. Stir it carefully.
5. Preheat the air fryer to 360 F.
6. Toss the butter in the air fryer basket and melt it.
7. After this, pour the apple sauce mixture into the melted almond butter.
8. Add the chopped smoked salmon.
9. Cook the omelet for 8 minutes.
10. Transfer the cooked omelet onto the serving plates.
11. Serve and enjoy!

Golden Cod Fish Nuggets

Servings: 4

Total Time: 25 Minutes

Calories: 168

Fat: 7.7 g

Protein: 16.8 g

Carbs: 0.4 g

Fiber: 1.2 g

Ingredients and Quantity

- 4 cod fillets
- 2 tbsp. olive oil
- 4 tbsp. apple sauce
- 1 cup breadcrumbs
- A pinch salt

Direction

1. Preheat the Air Fryer to 390 F.
2. Place the breadcrumbs, olive oil, and salt in a food processor and process until evenly combined.
3. Pour the breadcrumb mixture into a bowl, the apple sauce into another bowl, and the flour into a third bowl.
4. Toss the cod fillets in the flour, then in the apple sauce, and then in the breadcrumb mixture.
5. Place them in the fryer basket, close and cook for 9 minutes.
6. At the 5-minute mark, quickly turn the chicken nuggets over.
7. Once golden brown, remove onto a serving plate and serve with vegetable fries. Enjoy!

Full Baked Trout en Papillote with Herbs

Servings: 2

Total Time: 30 Minutes

Calories: 243

Fat: 8.1 g

Protein: 15.6 g

Carbs: 2.9 g

Fiber: 0.4 g

Ingredients and Quantity

- 3/4 lb. whole trout, scaled and cleaned
- 1/4 bulb fennel, sliced
- 1/2 brown onion, sliced
- 3 tbsp. chopped parsley
- 3 tbsp. chopped dill
- 2 tbsp. olive oil
- 1 lemon, sliced

- Salt and pepper, to taste

Direction

1. In a bowl, add the onion, parsley, dill, fennel, and garlic. Mix and drizzle the olive oil over.
2. Preheat the Air Fryer to 350 F.
3. Open the cavity of the fish and fill with the fennel mixture.
4. Wrap the fish completely in parchment paper and then in foil.
5. Place the fish in the fryer basket and cook for 10 minutes.
6. Remove the paper and foil, and top with lemon slices.
7. Serve with a side of cooked mushrooms. Enjoy!

Breaded Scallops

Servings: 6

Total Time: 5 Minutes

Calories: 280

Fat: 32 g

Protein: 2.8 g

Carbs: 3.2 g

Fiber: 0.5 g

Ingredients and Quantity

- 12 fresh scallops
- 3 tbsp. almond flour
- 4 salt and black pepper
- 3 tbsp. apple sauce
- 1 cup breadcrumbs

Direction

1. Coat the scallops with flour.
2. Dip into the apple sauce, then into the breadcrumbs.
3. Spray them with olive oil and arrange them in the air fryer.
4. Cook for 6 minutes at 360 F, turning once halfway through cooking. Serve and enjoy!

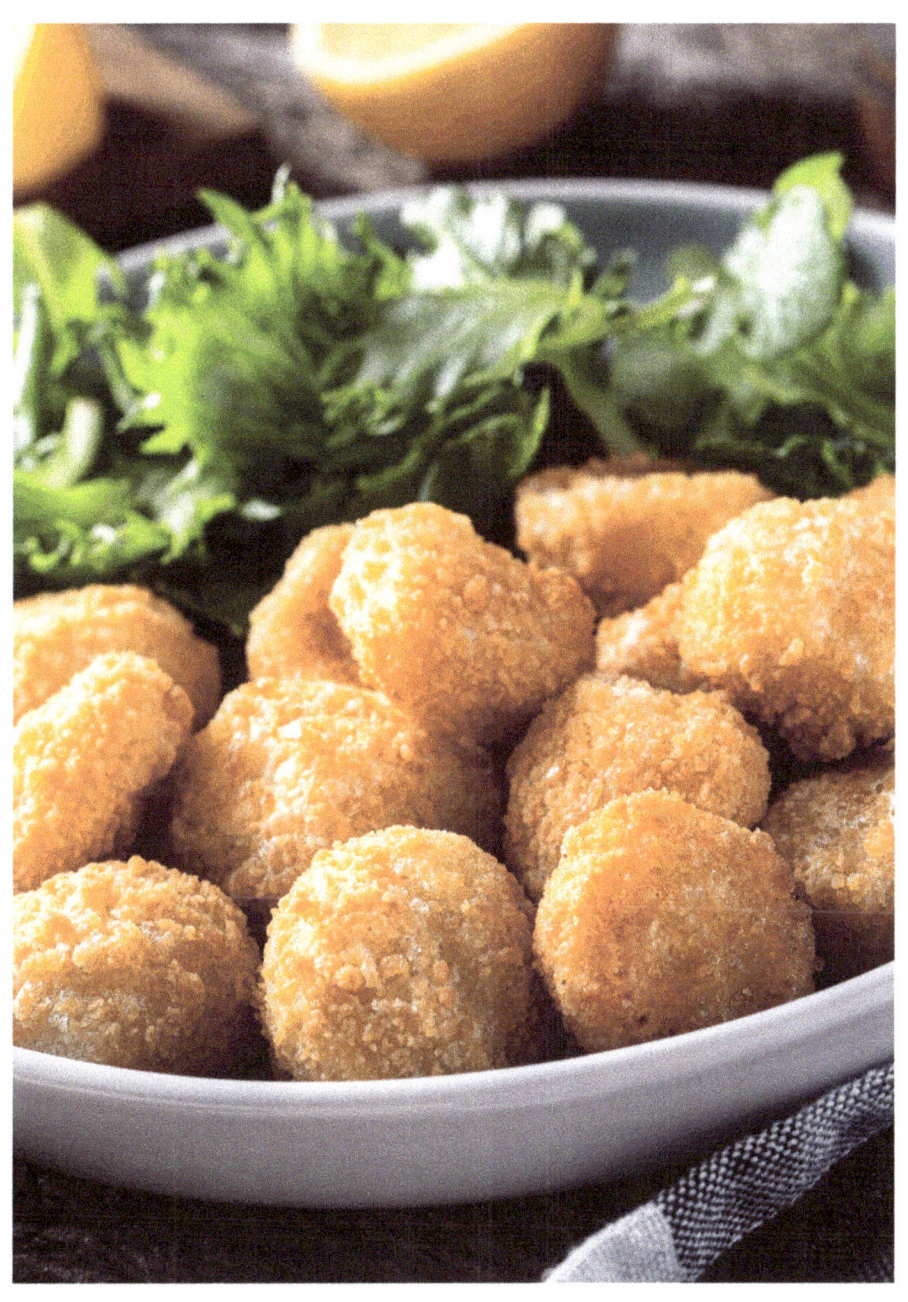

Hot Salmon and Broccoli

Servings: 2

Total Time: 25 Minutes

Calories: 368

Fat: 32 g

Protein: 4 g

Carbs: 5.8 g

Fiber: 3 g

Ingredients and Quantity

- 2 salmon fillets
- 1 tsp. olive oil
- Juice of 1 lime
- 1 tsp. chili flakes
- Salt and black pepper
- 1 head broccoli, cut into florets

- 1 tsp. olive oil
- 1 tbsp. soy sauce

Direction

1. In a bowl, add oil, lime juice, flakes, salt, and black pepper; rub the mixture onto fillets.
2. Lay the florets into your air fryer and drizzle with oil.
3. Arrange the fillets around or on top and cook at 340 F for 10 minutes.
4. Drizzle the florets with soy sauce to serve!

Soy Sauce Glazed Cod

Servings: 1

Total Time: 15 Minutes

Calories: 149

Fat: 5.8 g

Protein: 21 g

Carbs: 2.9 g

Fiber: 4 g

Ingredients and Quantity

- 1 cod fillet
- 1 tsp. olive oil
- A pinch sea salt
- A pinch pepper
- 1 tbsp. soy sauce
- Dash sesame oil

- 1/4 tsp. ginger powder
- 1/4 tsp. maple syrup

Direction

1. Preheat the Air fryer to 370 degrees.
2. Combine the olive oil, salt and pepper, and brush that mixture over the cod.
3. Place the cod onto an aluminum sheet and into the air fryer; cook for 6 minutes.
4. Meanwhile, combine the soy sauce, ginger, maple syrup, and sesame oil.
5. Brush the glaze over the cod.
6. Flip the fillet over and cook for 3 more minutes. Serve and enjoy!

County Baked Crab Cakes

Servings: 1

Total Time: 20 Minutes

Calories: 126

Fat: 5 g

Protein: 16 g

Carbs: 1.6 g

Fiber: 2 g

Ingredients and Quantity

- 1/2 pound jumbo crab
- Lemon juice, to taste
- 2 tbsp. parsley, chopped
- Old bay seasoning, as needed
- 1 tbsp. basil, chopped
- 3 tbsp. vegan mayo
- 1/4 tsp. Dijon mustard

- Zest of 1/2 lemo
- 1/4 cup panko breadcrumbs

Direction

1. Preheat your Fryer to 400 F, and in a bowl, mix mayo, lemon zest, old bay seasoning, mustard, and oil.
2. Blend crab meat in food processor and season with salt.
3. Transfer to the mixing bowl and combine well.
4. Form cakes using the mixture and dredge the mixture into breadcrumbs.
5. Place the cakes in your air fryer's basket and cook for 15 minutes.
6. Serve garnished with parsley and lemon juice. Enjoy!

Air Fried Salmon

Servings: 2

Total Time: 10 Minutes

Calories: 288

Fat: 19 g

Protein: 28 g

Carbs: 2 g

Fiber: 3 g

Ingredients and Quantity

- 2 wild caught salmon fillets with comparable thickness (about 1 1/12 inches thick)
- 2 tsp. avocado oil or olive oil
- 2 tsp. paprika
- Salt and coarse black pepper, to taste
- Lemon wedges

Direction

1. Remove any bones from your salmon (if necessary) and let fish sit on the counter for an hour.
2. Rub each fillet with olive oil and season with paprika, salt, and pepper.
3. Place fillets in the basket of the air fryer.
4. Set air fryer at 390 degrees for 7 minutes for 1½-inch fillets.
5. When timer goes off, open basket and check fillets with a fork to make sure they are done to your desired cook. Enjoy!

Air Fried Dragon Shrimp

Servings: 4

Total Time: 25 Minutes

Calories: 221

Fat: 13 g

Protein: 23 g

Carbs: 1 g

Fiber: 1.1 g

Ingredients and Quantity

- 1 pound raw shrimp, peeled and deveined 1/2 cup soy sauce
- 6 tbsp. apple sauce
- 2 tbsp. olive oil
- 1 cup yellow onion, diced
- 1/4 cup flour
- 1/2 tsp. red pepper, ground

- 1/2 tsp. ginger, grounded

Direction

1. Preheat your air fryer to 350 F.
2. Add all the ingredients except for the shrimp to make the batter.
3. Set it aside for 10 minutes.
4. Dip each shrimp into the batter to coat all sided.
5. Place them on the air fryer basket.
6. Cook for 10 minutes. Serve and enjoy!

Cheesy Haddock

Servings: 4

Total Time: 23 Minutes

Calories: 321

Fat: 15.7 g

Protein: 27.7 g

Carbs: 17 g

Ingredients and Quantity

- 4 haddock fillets
- 3/4 cup coconut milk
- 2 tsp. salt
- 3/4 cup bread crumbs
- 1/4 cup grated vegan cheese
- 1/4 tsp. ground dried thyme
- 1/4 cup almond butter, melted

Direction

1. Place in the ceramic pot the Foodi Cook and Crisp reversible rack.
2. Dip the haddock fillets in coconut milk then season with salt. Set aside.
3. In a mixing bowl, combine the bread crumbs, vegan cheese, and ground thyme.
4. Dredge the fillets in the bread crumbs mixture.
5. Place the fish on the reversible rack.
6. Brush withalmond butter on all sides.
7. Close the crisping lid and press the Bake/Roast button before pressing the Start button.
8. Adjust the cooking time to 20 minutes. Serve and enjoy!

Foil Baked Salmon

Servings: 2

Total Time: 23 Minutes

Calories: 619

Fat: 51.3 g

Protein: 36.3 g

Carbs: 2.9 g

Ingredients and Quantity

- 2 salmon fillets
- 2 garlic cloves, minced
- 6 tbsp. olive oil
- 1 tsp. dried basil
- 1 tsp. salt
- 1 tsp. ground black pepper
- 1 tbsp. lemon juice
- 1 tbsp. fresh parsley, chopped

Direction

1. Place in the ceramic pot the Foodi Cook and Crisp reversible rack.
2. On a large foil, place the salmon fillets and season with the rest of the ingredients.
3. Do not fold the aluminum foil.
4. Place the foil - fish and all - on the reversible tray.
5. Close the crisping lid and press the Bake/Roast button before pressing the START button.
6. Adjust the cooking time to 20 minutes or until the fish is flaky. Serve and enjoy!

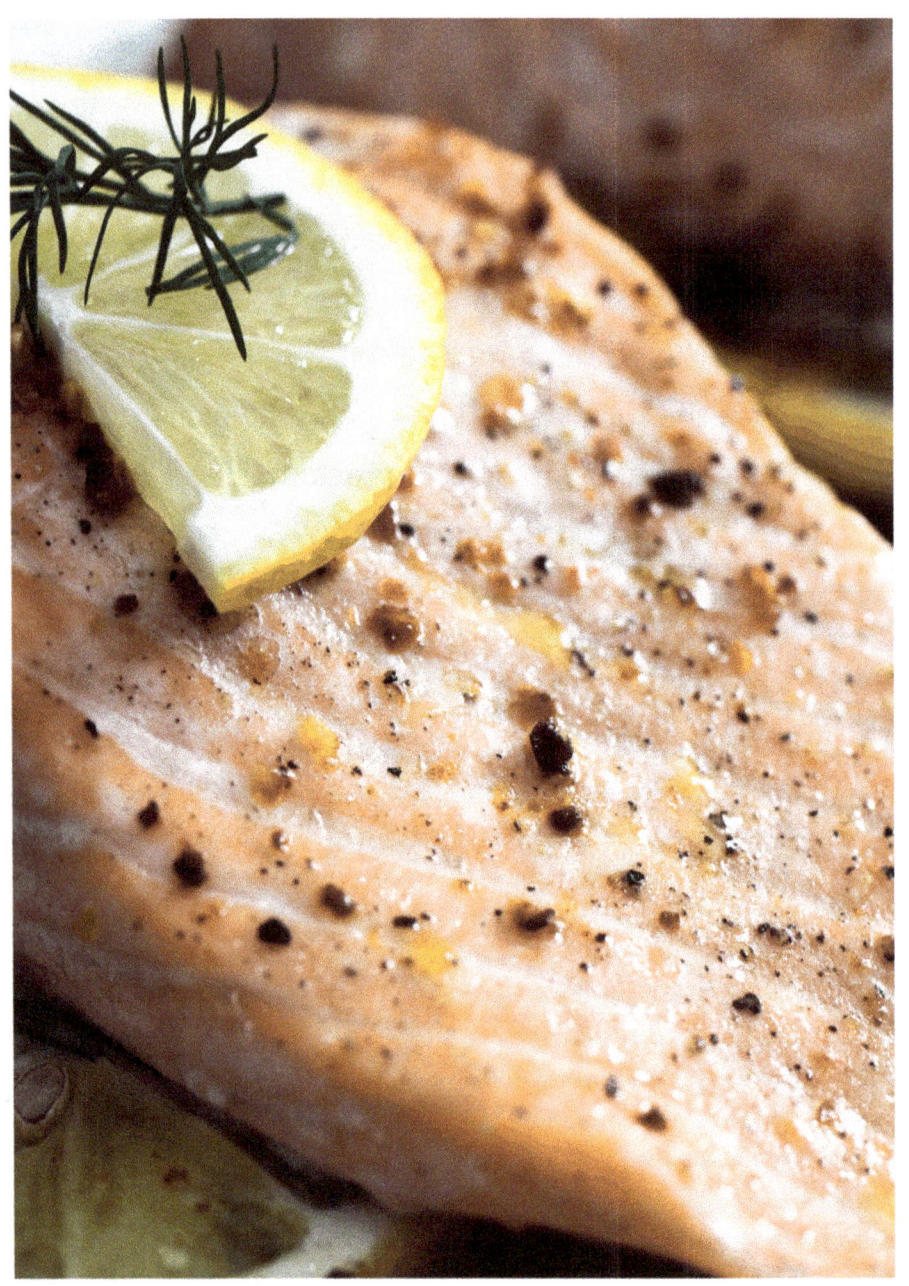

Pasta with Capers and Tuna

Servings: 4

Total Time: 25 Minutes

Ingredients and Quantity

- 1 tbsp. olive oil
- 1 garlic clove
- 3 anchovies
- 2 cups tomato puree
- 1 1/2 tsp. salt
- 16 oz. (500 g) fusilli pasta
- Two 5 1/2 oz. (160 g) cans Tuna packed in olive oil
- water to cover
- 2 tbsp. capers

Direction

1. In the pre-heated Foodi Multicooker on "Sauté" mode, add the oil, garlic and anchovies.
2. Sauté until the anchovies begin to disintegrate and the garlic cloves are just starting to turn golden.
3. Add the tomato puree and salt and mix together.
4. Pour in the uncooked pasta, and the contents of one tuna can (5 oz.) mixing to coat the dry pasta evenly.
5. Flatten the pasta in an even layer and pour in just enough water to cover.
6. Lock the lid on the Foodi Multicooker and then cook for 3 minutes. To get 3-minutes cook time, press "Pressure" button and use the Time Adjustment button to adjust the cook time to 3 minutes.
7. When time is up, open the cooker by releasing the pressure.
8. Mix in the last 5 oz. of tuna.
9. Close crisping lid and select Broil, set time to 7 minutes.

10. 10.Sprinkle with capers before serving.
Enjoy!

Tuna Bowls

Servings: 4

Total Time: 13 Minutes

Calories: 202

Fat: 7 g

Protein: 6 g

Carbs: 12 g

Fiber: 7 g

Ingredients and Quantity

- 16 oz. canned tuna, drained and flaked
- 1 red onion, chopped
- A handful baby spinach
- 1 tbsp. lime juice
- 2 spring onions, chopped
- 3 tbsp. butter, melted

Direction

1. Set the Foodi on Sauté mode, add the butter, heat it up, add the onion, stir and cook for 2 minutes.
2. Add the rest of the ingredients, toss.
3. Put the pressure lid on and cook on High for 5-6 minutes.
4. Release the pressure fast for 5 minutes.
5. Divide everything into bowls and serve. Enjoy!

Ranch Fish Fillet

Servings: 4

Total Time: 30 Minutes

Calories: 425

Fat: 25.4 g

Protein: 18.8 g

Carbs: 30.4 g

Ingredients and Quantity

- 3/4 cup bread crumbs
- 1 packet dry ranch dressing mix
- 2 1/2 tbsp. vegetable oil
- 6 tbsp. apple sauce
- fish fillets

Direction

1. Combine the bread crumbs and ranch mix in a bowl.
2. Pour in the oil.
3. Dip each fish fillet into the apple sauce and cover with the crumb mixture.
4. Place in the Ninja Foodi basket and seal the lid.
5. Select air crisp function.
6. Cook at 360 degrees F for 12 minutes, flipping halfway through.
7. You can garnish with lemon wedges. Enjoy!

Paprika Salmon

Servings: 2

Total Time: 25 Minutes

Calories: 248

Fat: 11.9 g

Protein: 34.9 g

Carbs: 1.5 g

Ingredients and Quantity

- 2 salmon fillets
- 2 tsp. avocado oil
- 2 tsp. paprika
- Salt and pepper, to taste

Direction

1. Coat the salmon with oil.

2. Season with salt, pepper and paprika.
3. Place in the Ninja Foodi basket.
4. Select the air crisp function.
5. Seal the crisping lid.
6. Cook at 390 degrees for 7 minutes.
7. You can garnish with lemon slices. Enjoy!

Fish Sticks

Servings: 2

Total Time: 25 Minutes

Calories: 549

Fat: 15 g

Protein: 61 g

Carbs: 39.4 g

Ingredients and Quantity

- 1 lb. cod, sliced into strips
- 1/2 cup tapioca starch
- 2 eggs
- 1 tsp. dried dill
- Salt and pepper, to taste
- 1 cup almond flour
- 1 tsp. onion powder
- 1/2 tsp. mustard powder

- 2 tbsp. avocado oil

Direction

1. Pat the cod fillet strips dry using paper towel.
2. Place the tapioca starch in a bowl.
3. In another bowl, beat the eggs.
4. In a larger bowl, mix the dill, salt, pepper, almond flour, onion powder and mustard powder.
5. Dip each strip in the first, second and third bowls.
6. Coat the Ninja Foodi basket with the avocado oil.
7. Place the fish strips inside. Cook at 390 degrees F for 5 minutes.
8. You can serve with tartar sauce. Enjoy!

Fish Fillet with Pesto Sauce

Servings: 3

Total Time: 28 Minutes

Calories: 383

Fat: 22.6 g

Protein: 42.1 g

Carbs: 2.2 g

Ingredients and Quantity

- 3 white fish fillets
- 1 tbsp. olive oil
- Salt and pepper, to taste
- 2 cups fresh basil leaves
- 2 garlic cloves, crushed
- 2 tbsp. pine nuts
- tbsp. vegan cheese, grated
- cup olive oil

Direction

1. Coat the fish fillets with 1 tablespoon of olive oil.
2. Season with the salt and pepper.
3. Place in the Ninja Foodi basket.
4. Cook at 320 degrees for 8 minutes.
5. While waiting, mix the remaining ingredients in a food processor.
6. Pulse until smooth.
7. Spread the pesto sauce on both sides of the fish before serving.
8. You can garnish with chopped pine nuts. Enjoy!

Hot Crispy Prawns

Servings: 4

Total Time: 25 Minutes

Calories: 490

Fat: 27.8 g

Protein: 0.3 g

Carbs: 8.7 g

Ingredients and Quantity

- 1 tsp. chili flakes
- 1 tsp. chili powder
- Salt and pepper, to taste
- 12 king prawns
- 3 tbsp. vegan mayonnaise
- 1 tbsp. ketchup
- 1 tbsp. wine vinegar

Direction

1. Combine all the spices in a bowl.
2. Toss the prawns in the spice mixture.
3. Place the prawns in the Ninja Foodi basket.
4. Seal the crisping lid.
5. Choose air crisp function.
6. Cook at 360 degrees for 8 minutes.
7. While waiting, mix the vegan mayo, ketchup and vinegar.
8. Serve with the prawns. Enjoy!

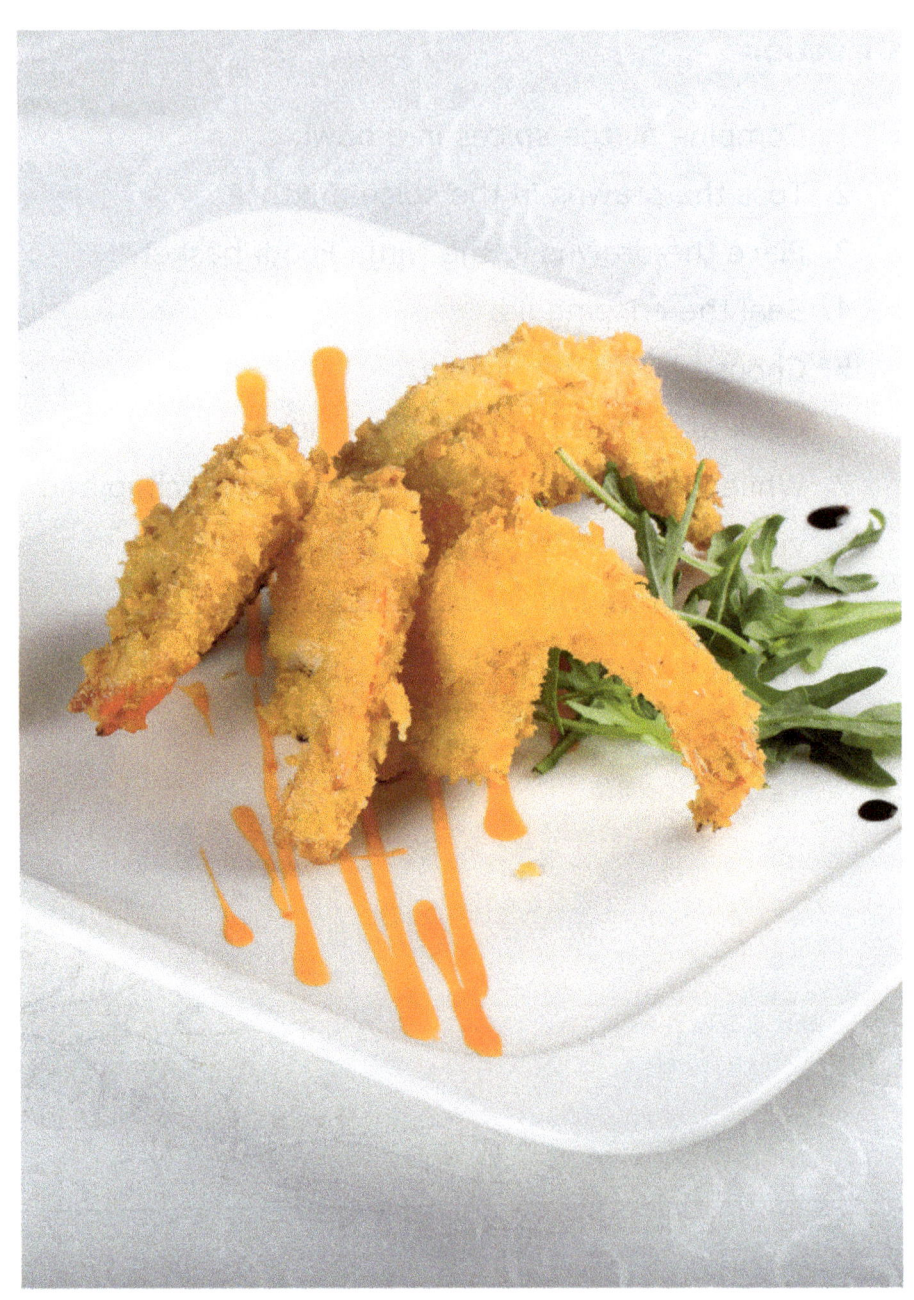

www.ingramcontent.com/pod-product-compliance
Lightning Source LLC
Chambersburg PA
CBHW070732030426
42336CB00013B/1947